Problem of Hair fall for women

Stress and Anxiety Scalp Health Medical Conditions and Hair Loss:

By
Ellie Grace

Table of contents

Introduction

Female going bald is a typical worry that can fundamentally affect a lady's confidence and personal satisfaction. While it is frequently connected with maturing, balding can influence ladies of any age and can be brought about by various elements. Grasping the causes, examples, and treatment choices for female going bald is fundamental for actually dealing with this condition and reestablishing certainty. In this exhaustive aide, we will investigate the different elements adding to female going bald, the various examples it can appear in, and the accessible treatment draws near.

Reasons for Female Going bald:

Hormonal Variables:

Hormonal irregular characteristics, for example, changes in estrogen and progesterone levels, can add to going bald in ladies.
Conditions like polycystic ovary condition (PCOS) and thyroid problems can likewise upset chemical levels and lead to hair diminishing.

Genetics:

Female example going bald, otherwise called androgen etic alopecia, can be acquired from one or the other parent and is described by a steady diminishing of hair on the scalp.
Dietary Lacks:

Insufficient admission of fundamental supplements, like iron, nutrients D and B12, and protein, can debilitate hair follicles and add to balding.

Stress and Uneasiness:

Profound pressure, uneasiness, and injury can set off a sort of balding called telegenic exhaust, where hair rashly enters the resting period of the hair development cycle and sheds more than expected.

Ailments:

Certain ailments, including immune system sicknesses like alopecia aerate and skin problems like lichen follicular can bring about balding in ladies.

Examples of Female Going bald:

Female Example Going bald (FPHL):

FPHL commonly presents as an enlarging part or diminishing along the highest point of the scalp, saving the hairline, and can advance to greater going bald over the long run.

Diffuse Hair Diminishing:

Diffuse hair diminishing is portrayed by a general reduction in hair thickness all through the scalp, with no unmistakable example of balding.

Sketchy Balding:

Sketchy going bald, as found in conditions like alopecia aerate, appears also characterized bare patches on the scalp or different region of the body.

Treatment Choices for Female Balding:

Skin Medicines:

Monoxide, a skin prescription, is FDA-endorsed for the treatment of FPHL and can advance hair development and forestall further misfortune when applied consistently to the scalp.

Oral Prescriptions:

Finasteride, an oral drug, might be endorsed off-mark for FPHL, however it isn't suggested for use in ladies of childbearing age because of potential birth surrenders. Nourishing Enhancements:

Supplements containing biotin, iron, zinc, and other fundamental supplements can assist with supporting sound hair development and forestall lacks that add to balding.

Platelet-Rich Plasma (PRP) Treatment:

PRP treatment includes infusing a concentrated arrangement of platelets from the patient's own blood into the scalp to invigorate hair follicle development and further develop hair thickness.

Hair Transplantation:

Hair transplantation systems, like follicular unit transplantation (FUT) and follicular unit extraction (FUE), can reestablish hair thickness by relocating sound hair follicles from giver destinations to diminishing or bare region of the scalp.

Conclusion:

Female going bald is a multifactorial condition that can fundamentally affect a lady's close to home prosperity and mental self portrait. By figuring out the fundamental causes, perceiving the examples of going bald, and investigating the accessible treatment choices, ladies can find proactive ways to address going bald and recapture trust in their appearance. Talking with a medical care proficient or dermatologist is fundamental for fostering a customized therapy plan custom-made to individual necessities and objectives. With the right methodology, ladies can really oversee balding and embrace sound, energetic hair indeed

Chapter 1
. Understanding Female Hair Loss

Going bald is frequently connected with men, yet it's a common issue for ladies too, influencing their actual appearance and close to home prosperity. Regardless of its commonness, female going bald remaining parts a point that is not examined as transparently as male balding. Figuring out the causes, medicines, and mental effects of female balding is vital for resolving this issue actually.

I. Sorts of Female Balding:

A. Androgen etic Alopecia:
1. Hereditary inclination
2. Hormonal elements
3. DHT responsiveness

B. Telligent Exhaust:
1. Stress-initiated balding
2. Pregnancy and labor
3. Drugs and ailments

C. Alopecia Aerate:
1. Immune system issue
2. Sets off and worsening variables
3. Mental stressors

D. Footing Alopecia:
1. Hairstyling rehearses
2. Tight hairdos
3. Social impacts

II. Reasons for Female Going bald:

A. Hormonal Irregular characteristics:
1. Menopause
2. Polycystic Ovary Condition (PCOS)
3. Thyroid issues

B. Healthful Inadequacies:
1. Lack of iron
2. Lack of vitamin D
3. Lack of protein

C. Ailments:
1. Lupus
2. Trichotillomania
3. Scalp contaminations

III. Medicines for Female Going bald:

A. Skin Medicines:
1. Monoxide (Rogaine)
2. Effective corticosteroids
3. Hair development serums

B. Oral Drugs:
1. Finasteride
2. Spironolactone
3. Oral contraceptives

C. Careful Intercessions:
1. Hair relocate a medical procedure
2. Scalp decrease a medical procedure

3. Platelet-rich plasma (PRP) treatment

D. Way of life Changes:
1. Dietary enhancements
2. Stress the executives strategies
3. Delicate hair care rehearses

IV. Mental Effects of Female Balding:

A. Self-perception Concerns:
1. Influence on confidence
2. Social withdrawal
3. Misery and tension

B. Methods for dealing with hardship or stress:
1. Support gatherings and guiding
2. Hairpiece and hairpiece use
3. Acknowledgment and confidence

C. Relationship Elements:
1. Accomplice and family support
2. Correspondence challenges
3. Closeness issues

V. Survival methods and Emotionally supportive networks:

A. Mental Help:
1. Treatment and directing
2. Care and unwinding strategies
3. Positive confirmations

B. Way of life Changes:
1. Solid eating regimen and exercise
2. Inventive articulation through design
3. Participating in leisure activities and interests

C. Local area Commitment:
1. Online gatherings and care groups
2. Nearby meatus and occasions
3. Backing and mindfulness crusades

End:

Female balding is a multi-layered issue impacted by hereditary, hormonal, ecological, and mental variables. Tending to female going bald requires a far reaching comprehension of its causes, medicines, and mental effects. By cultivating open exchange, giving successful medicines, and offering emotionally supportive networks, we can enable ladies to adapt to balding and embrace their excellence with certainty and flexibility.

Chapter 2

Hormonal Imbalance and Hair Loss:

Hormonal unevenness is a typical ailment that influences different parts of wellbeing, including hair development and misfortune. This article intends to investigate the association between hormonal lopsidedness and going bald, revealing insight into the components, causes, side effects, and accessible treatment choices.

Grasping Hormonal Awkwardness:

Chemicals are compound couriers that control various physical processes, including digestion, proliferation, development, and advancement. At the point when these chemicals are not delivered or managed appropriately, it can prompt a hormonal unevenness, upsetting the body's typical capabilities. Hormonal unevenness can happen because of different factors like hereditary qualities, maturing, stress, drugs, and basic ailments.

Chemicals and Hair Development Cycle:

Hair development follows a repetitive example comprising of three stages: antigen (development stage), cartage (momentary stage), and telegenic (resting stage). Chemicals assume a significant part in directing the hair development cycle. For instance, androgens, including testosterone and dihydrotestosterone (DHT), impact hair follicle movement and can either advance hair development or add to balding relying upon their levels and awareness in the body.

Impacts of Hormonal Unevenness on Hair:

Hormonal irregularity can upset the ordinary hair development cycle, prompting different hair-related issues, for example,

Telligent Exhaust

A condition described by over the top shedding of hair because of an unexpected hormonal lopsidedness, stress, disease, or wholesome lacks.

Androgen etic Alopecia:

Normally known as male or female example sparseness, it is an innate condition connected to hormonal irregular characteristics, especially the impacts of androgens on hair follicles.

Polycystic Ovary Condition (PCOS):

PCOS is a hormonal problem in ladies described by imbalanced degrees of androgens, insulin obstruction, and sporadic feminine cycles. One of the normal side effects of PCOS is male-design going bald or diminishing of scalp hair.

Thyroid Issues:

Both hypothyroidism and hyperthyroidism can disturb the hormonal equilibrium in the body, prompting going bald. Thyroid chemicals assume a crucial part in controlling digestion, which by implication influences hair development.

Conclusion of Hormonal Irregularity and Going bald:

Diagnosing hormonal lopsidedness and its relationship with going bald includes a thorough clinical assessment, including:

Clinical History:

An itemized survey of the patient's clinical history, including family background of going bald, hormonal problems, and other pertinent elements.

Actual Assessment: Assessment of the scalp, hair, and other actual elements to evaluate the example and seriousness of going bald.

Hormonal Testing:

Blood tests might be directed to quantify chemical levels, including testosterone, DHT, estrogen, progesterone, thyroid chemicals, and cortisol levels.

Scalp Biopsy: At times, a scalp biopsy might be performed to look at the hair follicles and decide any basic irregularities.

Treatment Choices for Hormonal Unevenness and Going bald:

The treatment approach for hormonal awkwardness and balding relies upon the fundamental reason and seriousness of the condition. Treatment choices might include:

Chemical Substitution Treatment (HRT): HRT includes enhancing lacking chemicals or managing chemical levels to reestablish harmony in the body. For instance, ladies with hormonal uneven characters because of menopause might profit from estrogen or progesterone substitution treatment.

Against androgen Prescriptions: Drugs that block the impacts of androgens, for example, Finasteride and spironolactone, might be endorsed to oversee androgen etic alopecia and other androgen-related going bald circumstances.

Skin Medicines: Monoxide, a skin medicine, is normally used to invigorate hair development and draw out the antigen period of the hair development cycle. It is available without a prescription and can be applied straightforwardly to the scalp.

Way of life Adjustments:

Embracing a sound way of life, including a reasonable eating regimen, customary activity, stress the executives strategies, and sufficient rest, can assist with supporting hormonal equilibrium and advance generally prosperity.

Careful Mediations:

In instances of cutting edge going bald or sparseness, careful choices, for example, hair transplantation might be considered to reestablish hair development and work on tasteful appearance.

Conclusion:

Hormonal irregularity can altogether affect hair development and lead to different types of going bald, including androgen etic alopecia, telegenic exhaust, and going bald related with hormonal problems like PCOS and thyroid issues. Understanding the hidden hormonal elements adding to balding is urgent for precise finding and viable treatment. By tending to hormonal awkward nature through fitting clinical mediations, way of life adjustments, and designated treatments, people encountering balding can further develop their hair wellbeing and in general personal satisfaction. Early location and mediation are vital to overseeing hormonal lopsidedness related going bald and accomplishing effective results.

Our hormones do a lot of work for us beyond making teenagers moody and distracted. Throughout our lives, hormones continue to perform vital functions for our overall health and well-being. But our bodies are imperfect machines and can either produce too many or too few of the hormones we need. These imbalances can throw normal processes out of whack, including the natural hair growth cycle.

Many cases of hair loss can be traced, in whole or in part, to hormone imbalances. Fortunately, medication and other treatments are available to restore balance to hormones and restore hair lost because of overactive or underactive hormone production.

How Do Hormones Affect Hair Growth and Loss?

Multiple hormones can impact the growth, strength, and health of our hair. The most common problems with hormone imbalances that can contribute to hair shedding and loss include:

A synthesized version of testosterone, DHT plays a role in sexual development and physical appearance. When too much testosterone gets converted into DHT, the natural growth cycle of hair is disrupted, causing hair follicle shrinkage or elimination and ultimately resulting in shedding or thinning hair.

Menopausal hair loss. Women going through menopause produce lower levels of estrogen and progesterone – two hormones critical for hair growth and follicle health. As these hormone levels decrease, hair growth slows while follicles become thin, brittle, and more vulnerable to damage. Making matters worse, the decrease in hair-promoting hormones is accompanied by an increase in androgens – hormones which trigger follicle miniaturization on the scalp. This miniaturization makes hair more susceptible to falling out.

Insulin Resistance. When the body fails to regulate insulin production properly, the body can build up a resistance to this hormone, which can, in turn, lead to an increased risk of androgen etic alopecia, or pattern baldness.

Medication and Other Treatments to Restore Balance and Restart Hair Growth

If you are experiencing hair loss and want to address the issue, the first step is identifying the causes behind the problem. Your physician plays an indispensable role in that process, including testing you for hormone and glucose imbalances. If you are indeed having trouble with hormone production, your doctor can prescribe medication which can help restore balance. Lifestyle changes, such as a healthier diet, exercise, and stress reduction will also help you get your hormone levels back on track.

Once equilibrium is restored to your hormones, hair loss associated with your hormone issue should slow or cease, and in many cases, hair that was loss may be replaced by new growth.

Additionally, many treatments we offer at the Hair Transplant Institute of Miami to treat other forms of hair loss are equally effective at addressing hair loss caused by hormonal imbalances. These can include hair transplant surgery, low-level laser therapy (LLLT), or hair loss medications.

Given the complications involved in hormone disorders and their treatment, only a consultation and full evaluation with an experienced hair loss physician can tell you which hair restoration treatment would be best for you.

Schedule an Appointment for a Hair Loss Evaluation Today

If a hormone imbalance is contributing to hair loss, the Hair Transplant Institute of Miami can help. We offer a range of effective treatments, customized to your individual condition

Chapter 3

Genetic Factors and Hair Loss

Going bald, restoratively known as alopecia, is a common concern influencing a great many individuals around the world. While different variables add to going bald, hereditary qualities assume a critical part in deciding a singular's helplessness to specific kinds of alopecia. This article digs into the complex connection between hereditary elements and going bald, investigating the components, legacy designs, risk variables, and progressions in hereditary examination pointed toward unwinding the secrets of genetic alopecia.

Grasping Genetic Alopecia:

Innate alopecia, likewise alluded to as hereditary balding or androgen etic alopecia, is the most widely recognized type of going bald, influencing all kinds of people. It is portrayed by a gradual diminishing of the hair, regularly beginning at the sanctuaries or crown of the scalp and step by step spreading to different regions. While the specific reason for genetic alopecia is multifactorial, hereditary inclination assumes an essential part in its turn of events.

Hereditary Systems of Going bald:

The legacy example of innate alopecia is complicated and includes various hereditary elements. One of the key givers is the communication between androgens (male chemicals) and hair follicles. Androgens, especially dihydrotestosterone (DHT), tie to androgen receptors in defenseless hair follicles, prompting scaling down of the follicles and possible hair diminishing and misfortune. Qualities associated with androgen digestion, follicle aversion to androgens, and hair follicle cycling are embroiled in the improvement of genetic alopecia.

Hereditary Gamble Variables for Inherited Alopecia:

A few hereditary gamble factors have been distinguished in relationship with genetic alopecia, including:

Androgen Receptor Quality (AR):

Varieties in the AR quality can impact the awareness of hair follicles to androgens, accordingly influencing the movement of androgen etic alopecia.

Qualities Associated with Hair Follicle Advancement and Cycling: Qualities answerable for directing hair follicle improvement, separation, and cycling can affect the weakness to genetic alopecia.

Polymorphisms in Chemical related Qualities: Hereditary varieties in qualities encoding chemicals, chemical receptors, and catalysts associated with chemical digestion can regulate the hormonal pathways ensnared in balding.

Legacy Examples of Innate Alopecia:

Innate alopecia displays a polygenic legacy design, implying that numerous qualities add to the gamble of fostering the condition. The legacy example can change contingent upon the particular qualities included and whether the condition is acquired from one or the two guardians. As a rule, innate alopecia will in general be more normal and extreme in people with a family background of the condition, recommending areas of strength for a part.

Hereditary Testing for Innate Alopecia:
Progressions in hereditary exploration have prompted the advancement of hereditary tests that can distinguish specific hereditary variations related with genetic alopecia. While hereditary testing for balding isn't yet generally accessible for clinical use, progressing research plans to work on how we might interpret the hereditary variables hidden alopecia and foster customized treatment approaches in light of hereditary profiling.

Hereditary Guiding and The executives of Innate Alopecia:

Hereditary guiding can assume a significant part in assisting people with understanding their gamble of genetic alopecia in light of family ancestry and hereditary inclination. Furthermore, early intercession and customized treatment methodologies can assist with dealing with the movement of balding and further develop results for people with inherited alopecia. Treatment choices might incorporate meds like monoxide and Finasteride, hair transplantation, and arising treatments focusing on unambiguous hereditary pathways associated with hair follicle guideline.

Hair loss or alopecia, a clinical condition that is frequently seen in dermatology clinics, can be caused by many etiological factors and it significantly affects the patients' quality of life [1]. This group of diseases is basically divided in two subgroups: cicatricle alopecia's and non-cicatricle alopecia's. While cicatricle alopecia may progress with loss of follicles, thus causing irreversible hair loss, this condition is usually reversible in non-cicatricle ones. Many causes are known to have a role in non-cicatricle alopecia, including emotional issues, chronic disorders, dietary inadequacies, trace elements, and vitamin deficiencies [2]. Other factors can be stress, drug use, immune system, endocrine disorders, and genetic and epigenetic changes [3].

A balanced and regular diet is very important for healthy hair: sudden weight loss, low-caloric diets, unbalanced diet, obesity, and excessive intake of vitamin and mineral supplements can cause hair loss. Micronutrients, which are the main elements of the hair follicle cycle, are very important in alopecia, which is why dietary supplements (mostly vitamin and mineral) are among the preferred methods to prevent hair loss. Given the frequency of hair loss in current times and its impact on the patients' social lives, finding effective alopecia treatments impacts a huge portion of the population [2].

The role of diet in the development and treatment of alopecia has recently been a hot topic of research. It has been found that plant-rich diets – such as the Mediterranean Diet (MD), whose main nutrients are rich in antioxidants, anti-inflammatory, and estrogenic components – include chemicals that stimulate hair growth and reduce hair loss. These diets contain phytochemicals that promote hair development by lowering the generation of reactive oxygen species in the dermal papilla cells, causing growth hormones to be secreted [4].

This is why dietary practices characterized by a large intake of anti-inflammatory, antioxidant and estrogenic activities are emphasized as additional treatments for alopecia. This review aims to explain the general background of alopecia, to emphasize the role of nutritional and dietary supplements in the treatment of alopecia, and to consider the effects of herbal treatment methods on alopecia patients.

Go to:
Alopecia and types of alopecia

Alopecia is the partial or complete loss of hair, which can be caused by a disruption in the hair development cycle or by damage to the hair follicles as a result of systemic or local factors such as genetics, hormone imbalances, and infection [5-7].

The hair growth cycle consists of four stages

: the antigen phase (the growth phase, which is also the longest, lasting 2-7 years); the cartage phase (the transitional phase, lasting up to 2 weeks, which includes hair follicle involution due to apoptosis); the telegenic phase (the resting phase, lasting up to 12 weeks); and the exogenous phase (the release phase of telegenic hair) [8].

The fact that alopecia is affected by many factors causes the existence of a wide number of types of alopecia. Androgenic alopecia, alopecia aerate, chemotherapy-induced alopecia, antigen effluvium, telegenic effluvium, traction alopecia, and trichotillomania are some of the most common kinds. The clinical classification system of Rook and Dauber divides all types of alopecia into two categories: cicatricle alopecia and non-cicatricle alopecia [6, 7].

CICATRICIAL ALOPECIAS

Cicatricle alopecia's (CAs) are clinical pathological conditions that describe permanent hair loss caused by the replacement of damaged hair follicles with fibrotic scar tissue. They are classified into two groups, primary cicatricle alopecia (PCA) and secondary cicatricle alopecia (SCA) [9, 10].

The PCA group includes multiple inflammatory diseases with distinct clinical and histopathological features and unknown and irreversible causes, primarily affecting and destroying hair follicles. It is responsible for 7% of all hair loss cases. PCA is subdivided into lymphocytic, neutrophil, or mixed subtypes [11, 12]. Chronic cutaneous lupus erythematous, lichen follicular classic Brooch pseudopelade, folliculitis decal vans, and dissection folliculitis are some of the diseases with clinical conditions [13].

The SCA group includes inflammatory and neoplastic conditions and physical traumas that usually affect primarily the dermis and cause secondary follicular destruction [9]. While in PCAs the disease directly affects hair follicles, in SCAs they disappear due to secondary reasons. Factors affecting SCA formation include genodermatoses, permanent alopecia due to developmental defects, physical and chemical injuries, infections, inflammatory dermatomes, drug uses, and neoplastic conditions

Chapter 4

Nutritional Deficiencies and Hair Fall:

Going bald, restoratively known as alopecia, is a common concern influencing a large number of individuals around the world. While different elements add to going bald, hereditary qualities assume a huge part in deciding a singular's defenselessness to specific sorts of alopecia. This article digs into the many-sided connection between hereditary variables and balding, investigating the systems, legacy designs, risk elements, and headways in hereditary examination pointed toward unwinding the secrets of genetic alopecia.

Figuring out Genetic Alopecia:

Innate alopecia, likewise alluded to as hereditary going bald or androgen etic alopecia, is the most widely recognized type of balding, influencing all kinds of people. It is portrayed by a gradual diminishing of the hair, normally beginning at the sanctuaries or crown of the scalp and step by step spreading to different regions. While the specific reason for genetic alopecia is multifactorial, hereditary inclination assumes a vital part in its turn of events.

Hereditary Components of Balding:

The legacy example of inherited alopecia is intricate and includes different hereditary variables. One of the key donors is the cooperation between androgens (male chemicals) and hair follicles. Androgens, especially dihydrotestosterone (DHT), tie to androgen receptors in vulnerable hair follicles, prompting scaling down of the follicles and possible hair diminishing and misfortune. Qualities engaged with androgen digestion, follicle aversion to androgens, and hair follicle cycling are embroiled in the improvement of genetic alopecia.

Hereditary Gamble Variables for Inherited Alopecia:

A few hereditary gamble factors have been recognized in relationship with genetic alopecia, including:

Androgen Receptor Quality (AR): Varieties in the AR quality can impact the responsiveness of hair follicles to androgens, consequently influencing the movement of androgen etic alopecia.

Qualities Engaged with Hair Follicle Advancement and Cycling: Qualities answerable for managing hair follicle improvement, separation, and cycling can influence the weakness to inherited alopecia.

Polymorphisms in Chemical related Qualities: Hereditary varieties in qualities encoding chemicals, chemical receptors, and catalysts engaged with chemical digestion can regulate the hormonal pathways embroiled in going bald.

Legacy Examples of Innate Alopecia:

Genetic alopecia displays a polygenic legacy design, implying that different qualities add to the gamble of fostering the condition. The legacy example can fluctuate contingent upon the particular qualities included and whether the condition is acquired from one or the two guardians. As a general rule, genetic alopecia will in general be more normal and serious in people with a family background of the condition, recommending areas of strength for a part.

Hereditary Testing for Inherited Alopecia:

Headways in hereditary examination have prompted the advancement of hereditary tests that can distinguish specific hereditary variations related with genetic alopecia. While hereditary testing for going bald isn't yet generally accessible for clinical use, continuous examination plans to work on how we might interpret the hereditary variables hidden alopecia and foster customized treatment approaches in light of hereditary profiling.

Hereditary Directing and The executives of Inherited Alopecia:

Hereditary directing can assume a significant part in assisting people with understanding their gamble of innate alopecia in view of family ancestry and hereditary inclination. Furthermore, early mediation and customized treatment procedures can assist with dealing with the movement of going bald and further develop results for people with genetic alopecia. Treatment choices might incorporate drugs like monoxide and Finasteride, hair transplantation, and arising treatments focusing on unambiguous hereditary pathways engaged with hair follicle guideline.

Future Headings in Hereditary Exploration on Going bald:

As our insight into the hereditary premise of going bald keeps on extending, future examination endeavors are centered around:

Distinguishing novel hereditary markers related with genetic alopecia.

Creating prescient models to evaluate individual gamble of balding in view of hereditary elements.

Investigating designated treatments that tweak hereditary pathways embroiled in hair follicle capability and guideline.

Improving hereditary testing innovations for precise determination and customized treatment arranging.

Conclusion:

Hereditary variables assume a critical part in the turn of events and movement of genetic alopecia, the most well-known type of balding. Understanding the hereditary instruments hidden alopecia can illuminate analytic methodologies, customized treatment techniques, and hereditary guiding for impacted people. Continuous headways in hereditary examination hold guarantee for unwinding the intricacies of genetic alopecia and further developing results for those impacted by this condition. By coordinating hereditary experiences into clinical practice, we can make ready for more powerful administration and avoidance of genetic going bald from now on.

Patients with hair loss often inquire whether nutritional supplements can help restore hair growth or prevent further hair loss. In fact, many will start dietary supplements without consultation in the hope that the supplements will help. The unregulated supplement industry also capitalizes on this population's vulnerability. While hair follicles are among the most metabolically active in the body, and hair growth may be impacted by calorie and protein malnutrition as well as micronutrient deficiency, the links are complex.

Nutritional deficiency may impact both hair structure and hair growth. Effects on hair growth include acute telegenic effluvium (TE), a well-known effect of sudden weight loss or decreased protein intake [1], as well as the diffuse alopecia seen in niacin deficiency [2]. Studies have also reported potential associations between nutritional deficiency and chronic TE, androgen etic alopecia (AGA), female pattern hair loss (FPHL), and alopecia aerate (AA) [3,4].

Given this well-recognized link, many patients seeking treatment for hair loss ask about dietary recommendations. Specifically, is it necessary to test for nutrient deficiency in a patient presenting with hair loss? Are there risk factors that should prompt testing? In the absence of such risk factors, is there any evidence to support the use of micronutrient supplementation?

Physicians must be prepared to answer these questions. Hair loss is common, with close to 50% of men and women affected by pattern hair loss by age 50 [5]. Many nutritional supplements are marketed as hair loss treatments. A search of the keywords "hair loss" within the Vitamins & Dietary Supplements section of Amazon.com, which sells supplements via Internet sales, yields 923 products [6]. Many are composed of differing formulations. The U.S. Food and Drug Administration (FDA) does not have the authority to review dietary supplements for safety and effectiveness before they are marketed, and it is therefore the responsibility of manufacturers [7].

Given the marketing efforts directed to consumers, physicians must be able to respond with a review of the known evidence. One point to emphasize is that such supplements are not without risks. In the absence of deficiency, supplementation may actually prove harmful to hair. Over-supplementation of certain nutrients, including selenium, Vitamin A, and Vitamin E, has actually been linked to hair loss [4,8–11]. It is therefore surprising that the best-selling hair supplement on Amazon.com contains both vitamin A and vitamin E [12], while the next contains selenium, vitamin A, and vitamin E [13].

While such products contain a variety of nutrients, review of the medical literature finds a notable lack of evidence supporting their use. Much of what is known about nutrient effect on hair loss is based on disease states that result in deficiency. There is currently a lack of literature regarding the effects of supplementation in individuals without nutrient deficiency. In this paper, we review the available literature on nutrient deficiencies that result in hair loss, detail the risk factors for these deficiencies, and review the available evidence of the effects of supplementation, both beneficial and adverse, on hair loss.

Go to:
Iron

Iron deficiency (ID) is the world's most common nutritional deficiency and is a well-known cause of hair loss. What remains unclear is what degree of ID may contribute to hair loss.

While the mechanism of action by which iron impacts hair growth is not known, hair follicle matrix cells are some of the most rapidly dividing cells in the body, and ID may contribute to hair loss via its role as a cofactor for rib nucleotide reeducates, the rate-limiting enzyme for DNA synthesis [14]. In addition, multiple genes have been identified in the human hair follicle [15], and some may be regulated by iron [16]. In a mouse model, reversal of ID led to restoration of hair growth [17].

Certain populations are at higher risk for ID, and a medical and dietary history may reveal risk factors. Premenopausal women are at higher risk due to menstrual blood loss, while postmenopausal women and men may present due to gastrointestinal blood loss. Other risk factors include malabsorption disorders (such as celiac disease) as well as achlorhydria or the use of H2 blockers, as iron requires an acidic pH for absorption.

Vegans and vegetarians are also at higher risk for ID, as their requirements for dietary iron are considered to be 1.8 times higher than for meat consumers [18]. Non-home iron, found in plants, has a lower bioavailability than home iron, found in meat and fish [19].

Patients with more advanced ID develop iron deficiency anemia and require replacement. ID may also result in a reduction of storage iron, measured by serum ferritin. A normal ferritin level does not exclude ID, however, as it is an acute phase reactant.

Although multiple research studies have been conducted, it is unknown if a deficiency of storage iron contributes to hair loss, as conflicting results have been noted. Some studies have found that low serum ferritin is more prevalent in patients with chronic TE, FPHL, AGA, and AA. Other studies have found no such link. Two excellent review articles have summarized these results and note considerable variations in study design, controls, and ID definitions [16,20]. There are few intervention trials, and they are limited by small numbers, lack of controls in some, and variable ferritin levels. These have utilized different interventions, including iron alone [21], iron with L-lysine [8,22], and iron with spironolactone [23].

One study used a control population that excluded patients at risk for ID [24] and found no statistically significant increase in the prevalence of ID in premenopausal or postmenopausal women with chronic TE or FPHL.

At this time, there are no definitive answers. Patients must be approached on a case-by-case basis. In the aforementioned review articles, the researchers present their approach. Both groups test patients with iron studies, including serum ferritin. Both recommend treatment of ID, with or without anemia, with dietary sources and oral iron supplementation when necessary, with a goal of ferritin levels above 50 mg/L [16] or 70 mg/ml, respectively [20].

Patients are monitored to measure their response—an important point. Patients who take iron supplements without monitoring are at risk for potentially severe complications, as iron supplementation leading to iron overload can cause toxicity. This can occur even at low levels if taken over a long period [25].

Go to:
Zinc
Zinc is an essential mineral required by hundreds of enzymes and multiple transcription factors that regulate gene expression [26]. While the exact

mechanism of action is unclear, one possibility centers on zinc's role as an essential component of numerous metalloenzymes important in protein synthesis and cell division [27]. Another possibility is zinc's role in the Hedgehog signaling pathway [28], a critical component in the pathways that govern hair follicle morphogenesis [29].

Zinc deficiency may be either inherited or acquired and may affect multiple organ systems. Patients may experience diarrhea, immunological effects, and delayed wound healing. Abnormalities in taste and smell may occur. Cutaneous effects include accrual and periorificial dermatitis, while hair changes include TE and brittle hair.

The autosomal recessive disorder, acrodermatitis thesaurus results in decreased absorption of zinc, while acquired zinc deficiency may occur in malabsorption syndromes, such as inflammatory bowel disease [30] or following gastric bypass surgery. Other groups at risk include patients with malignancy, those with liver or renal dysfunction, pregnant women [31], and patients with alcoholism [32]. Drugs that can affect zinc levels include valproic acid [33] and certain antihypertensive [34].

Dietary risk factors include vegetarianism, as bioavailability of zinc is lower in vegetables than meat [35]. Additionally, vegetarians typically consume more legumes and whole grains, which contain phytates that bind to zinc and inhibit absorption [35].

Serum zinc, the most commonly measured index of zinc status, may be impacted by several variables, and the functional effects of deficiency may be observed before serum levels decrease below normal [36].

Screening in those with risk factors is indicated, as hair loss due to zinc deficiency can be reversed. A case series demonstrated reversal of hair loss following oral supplementation in five patients with TE and zinc deficiency [37].

A study of 312 patients with AA, male pattern hair loss (MPHL), FPHL, or TE showed that all groups had statistically lower zinc concentrations as compared to 30 healthy controls [38]. In patients with AA and low serum zinc levels, supplementation has been shown to have therapeutic effects [39].

However, there is currently limited information on the effects of zinc supplementation on hair growth in those without documented deficiency. One report described a single patient with alopecia, without clear deficiency, who experienced improvement following oral zinc therapy [40].

A major point when considering supplementation in the absence of known deficiency is that zinc toxicity can occur with excess supplementation. Acute adverse effects include pain, vomiting, and diarrhea, while chronic effects include interaction with iron and reduced immune function [18].

Go to:
Niacin

Pellagra, due to a deficiency of niacin, results in the well-known triad of photosensitive dermatitis, diarrhea, and dementia. Alopecia is another frequent clinical finding [2].

Pellagra became rare in many developed countries after niacin fortification of food was introduced. Alcoholism is now considered the most common cause of pellagra in developed countries [41]. Other causes include malabsorption disorders or drug-induced cases, such as with isoniazid [41].

In a review of the literature, no studies regarding niacin levels in patients presenting only with hair loss were identified.

Go to:
Fatty Acids

Deficiency of the polyunsaturated essential fatty acids linoleic acid (an omega-6 fatty acid) and alpha-linoleic acid (an omega-3 fatty acid) can result from inappropriate parenteral nutrition and malabsorption disorders such as cystic fibrosis. Hair changes include loss of scalp hair and eyebrows as well as lightening of hair [3,4]. Unsaturated fatty acids may modulate androgen action by inhibition of 5α-reeducates, similar to the drug Finasteride [42]. Additionally, arachidonic acid, an omega-6 fatty acid, may promote hair growth by enhancing follicle proliferation [43].

However, limited information is available on supplementation. In one patient with essential fatty acid deficiency, topical application of safflower oil, high in linoleic acid, resulted in growth of hair [44].

While results from a trial utilizing a supplement were reported, limited conclusions may be drawn, as this supplement combined multiple fatty acids and antioxidants [45].

Go to:
Selenium

Selenium is an essential trace element that plays a role in protection from oxidative damage as well as hair follicle morphogenesis. Rats deficient in selenium display sparse hair growth [46], while knockout mice lacking specific selenoproteins exhibit progressive hair loss after birth [47].

Risk factors for deficiency include living in areas with low selenium soil content (particularly in parts of China, Tibet, and Siberia), long-term hemodialysis, HIV, and malabsorption disorders [48].

There is limited research on selenium deficiency and alopecia in humans. One case report in a child described sparse hair, which improved after dietary supplementation [49].

Given the lack of human research, it is surprising that some hair loss supplements are marketed as containing selenium. This is concerning, as selenium toxicity from nutritional supplementation is well documented [9–11]. Toxicity can result in generalized hair loss, as well as blistering skin lesions, gastrointestinal symptoms, and memory difficulties.

Go to:
Vitamin D

Data from animal studies suggests that vitamin D plays a role in hair follicle cycling [50]. In a study of mice treated to model vitamin D-dependent rickets, the resultant animals developed hair loss [51]. In vitro studies have shown increase in vitamin D receptor expression in the outer root sheath keratinocytes during the growing phases of the hair cycle [52].

Risk factors for vitamin D deficiency include inadequate sun exposure, dark skin, obesity, gastric bypass, and fat malabsorption [53].

One study of eight females with TE or FPHL showed that serum vitamin D2 levels were significantly lower than in controls. Furthermore, vitamin D2 levels decreased with increased disease severity [54]. However, data on the effects of vitamin D supplementation in hair loss is lacking.

Go to:
Vitamin A

Vitamin A is a group of compounds including retinol, retinal, retinoic acid, and provitamin A carotenoids. In murine studies, dietary vitamin A has been shown to activate hair follicle stem cells [55], although its role is recognized as complex and "precise levels of retinoic acid are needed for optimal function of the hair follicle" [56].

While deficiency has not been linked to hair loss, high levels of vitamin A have. In fact, one study found that in a mouse AA model, reduction of vitamin A in the diet actually delayed hair loss onset [56].

In humans, hypervitaminosis A may result from over-supplementation and has a strong known link to hair loss with other effects such as skin, vision, and bone changes [4,8].

Go to:
Vitamin E

Tocotrienols and tocopherols are members of the vitamin E family and are potent antioxidants. Deficiency results in hemolytic anemia's, neurologic findings, and skin dryness. Vitamin E deficiency is rare, but may occur with fat malabsorption disorders.

Minimal information in the literature exists regarding benefits of vitamin E supplementation on hair loss. One study of 21 volunteers who received Tocotrienols supplementation (100 mg of mixed Tocotrienols daily) showed significant increase in hair number as compared to a placebo group [57].

However, excess supplementation may result in hypervitaminosis E, which can increase the risk of bleeding and decrease thyroid hormone production. Additionally, there is some evidence for an adverse effect on hair growth, as seen in volunteers taking 600 IU per day for 28 days, a dosage around 30 times the daily recommended intake [8]. This group had significant decreases in thyroid hormone levels [8].

Go to:
Folic Acid

Folic acid is found in leafy greens and many foods are fortified with folic acid, making deficiency uncommon. Deficiency mainly results in megaloblastic anemia, without manifestation of hair loss.

No significant difference in serum foliate levels was seen in 91 patients with diffuse hair loss as compared to controls [58]. In fact, another study of 200 women with chronic TE showed 28.5% had elevated serum folic acid, although methodology of the study was not included and therefore limited conclusions may be drawn [8].

Go to:
Biotin

Biotin, or vitamin H, serves as a cofactor for carboxylation enzymes. In isolated sheep hair follicles, incubation in biotin-containing solutions resulted in increased DNA concentration and protein synthesis [59].

Symptoms of deficiency include eczematous skin rash, alopecia, and conjunctivitis [60]. One study of an infant fed with a formula lacking sufficient biotin content reported manifestations of periorificial dermatitis and patchy alopecia, both of which resolved with daily oral supplementation of biotin [61].

Biotin deficiency is rare, as intestinal bacteria are typically able to produce adequate levels of biotin. Deficiency is seen in cases of congenital or acquired biotinidase or carboxylase deficiency, antibiotic use disrupting the gastrointestinal flora, and antiepileptic use. Deficiency can occur from excessive ingestion of raw egg whites due to binding by avid in.

No clinical trials have shown efficacy in treating hair loss with biotin supplementation in the absence of deficiency. Despite this, biotin is found in multiple supplements marketed to consumers for hair loss. This marketing approach may have been chosen as biotin has shown positive effects in the treatment of brittle fingernails and onychoschizia [62–63].

Go to:
Amino Acids and Proteins
Protein malnutrition, such as in kwashiorkor and marasmus, can result in hair changes that include hair thinning and hair loss [64].

One study examined the role of L-lysine, an essential amino acid that may play a role in iron and zinc uptake. Addition of L-lysine to iron supplementation resulted in a significant increase in mean serum ferritin concentration in some women with chronic TE who failed to respond to iron supplementation alone [8]. Although interesting, there is limited data available, and \the role of L-lysine should be investigated further.

In terms of other amino acids and proteins, no clear conclusions may be drawn about the role of supplementation in hair loss. While trials of amino acid and protein supplements have been published, they are formulated with a variety of nutrients, and therefore it is unclear what role, if any, is played by amino acid and protein supplementation in the absence of known deficiency.

One trial included L-cysteine, a constituent of keratin, in combination with medicinal yeast and pantothenic acid [65]. Other trials have evaluated supplements containing marine proteins in conjunction with multiple other nutrients [66–69]. However, it is difficult to evaluate the results of these trials, as the composition of these nutritional supplements is not disclosed. Marketing materials accessed from one product's website describe the composition as including "vitamins and minerals for hair growth, including iron, zinc, biotin, niacin, vitamin C and an exclusive marine complex derived from fish proteins" [70].

Go to:
Antioxidants

Antioxidants are compounds that are able to neutralize reactive oxygen species (ROS), preventing oxidative damage. Many substances can be classified as antioxidants, including zinc, selenium, and vitamins A and E, as described previously in this article, as well as vitamin C and polyphenols [71]. Oxidative stress has been linked to hair loss. In vitro studies of dermal papilla cells from male AGA patients have shown that oxidative stress may have an important role in the balding phenotype and development of AGA [72]. Additionally, in a study of endogenous antioxidant enzymes and lipid peroxidation in the scalps of patients with AA, excessive free radical generation was shown to occur in the scalps of patients with AA accompanied by high levels of antioxidant enzymes that were unable to protect against the ROS [73].

While dietary antioxidants play a key role in reinforcing our endogenous antioxidant system, high doses of exogenous antioxidants may actually disrupt the balance between oxidation and ant oxidation [71]. In vitro studies have shown that while polyphenols have antioxidant properties at low concentrations, they can potentiate ROS generation at higher concentrations [71, 74–75]. Compounds within plant foods, such as from fruits, vegetables, and grains, may be safer and healthier compared to isolated, high doses present in supplements [71].

Go to:

Conclusion

While multiple nutrient deficiencies may result in hair loss (Table 1), screening for such deficiencies must be guided by the history and physical exam. Nutrient deficiencies may arise due to genetic disorders, medical conditions, or dietary practices.

Chapter 5

Stress, Anxiety, and Hair Loss

Stress and uneasiness are normal encounters in the present high speed world, influencing a large number of individuals around the world. While intermittent pressure is a typical piece of life, persistent pressure and tension can unfavorably affect both physical and psychological wellness. One of the less popular outcomes of constant pressure and tension is going bald. This paper plans to investigate the many-sided connection between stress, uneasiness, and going bald, including their causes, impacts, and the executives methodologies.

I. Figuring out Pressure and Tension:

A. Definition and Kinds of Stress:

Stress as the body's reaction to requests or tensions.
Qualification among intense and ongoing pressure.
B. Definition and Sorts of Nervousness:

Tension as a determined sensation of stress, dread, or disquiet.
Various sorts of tension issues, including summed up nervousness jumble (Stray), alarm turmoil, and social uneasiness problem.

II. The Physiology of Stress and Uneasiness:

A. The Job of Pressure Chemicals:

Cortisol:
 The essential pressure chemical and its consequences for the body.
Adrenaline: The "survival" chemical and its momentary impacts.

B. The Effect of Constant Pressure and Uneasiness:

Drawn out rise of cortisol levels and its adverse consequences on different substantial frameworks.
The connection between ongoing pressure/tension and cardiovascular sicknesses, stomach related issues, and invulnerable concealment.

III. Figuring out Balding:

A. Ordinary Hair Development Cycle:

Anlagen stage: Development period of hair follicles.
Cartagena stage: Momentary stage.
Telligent stage: Resting stage before hair shedding.

B. Kinds of Balding:

Androgen etic Alopecia (Male and Female Example Hairlessness).
telegenic Exhaust: Stress-actuated hair shedding.
Alopecia Aerate: Immune system related going bald.
IV. The Connection Between Stress, Uneasiness, and Balding:

A. Components of Stress-Prompted Balding:

Telligent Emanation:

Disturbance of the hair development cycle because of stress.
Neuroendocrine Variables: Effect of pressure chemicals on hair follicles.
B. Research Concentrates on Pressure Instigated Going bald:

Clinical investigations connecting ongoing pressure and going bald.
Mental elements adding to balding movement.
V. Overseeing Pressure and Uneasiness to Forestall Balding:

A. Stress The board Strategies:

Care Contemplation.
Profound Breathing Activities.
Yoga and Kendo.

B. Mental Intercessions:

Mental Social Treatment (CBT) for uneasiness issues.
Stress-decrease methods in psychotherapy.

C. Way of life Alterations:

Standard Activity.
Solid Eating routine plentiful in nutrients and minerals fundamental for hair wellbeing.
VI. Treatment Choices for Stress-Incited Going bald:

A. Skin Medicines:

Monoxide:
Non-prescription drug to advance hair development.
Supplement rich serums and oils.

B. Oral Drugs:

Finasteride: Professionally prescribed prescription for androgen etic alopecia.
Supplements like biotin and iron for generally hair wellbeing.

C. High level Medicines:

Platelet-Rich Plasma (PRP) Treatment.
Low-level Laser Treatment (LLLT).

VII. Conclusion:

Ongoing pressure and nervousness can fundamentally affect hair wellbeing, prompting conditions like telegenic exhaust and worsening existing balding circumstances. Understanding the physiological components behind pressure prompted balding is vital for creating compelling administration and treatment procedures. By executing pressure decrease methods, mental intercessions, and suitable hair care rehearses, people can moderate the impacts of pressure and uneasiness on their hair and generally speaking prosperity.

VIII. References:

[Rundown of scholarly papers, research studies, and legitimate sources supporting the data introduced in the paper.]

This exhaustive investigation of the connection between stress, uneasiness, and balding gives significant bits of knowledge into the mind boggling exchange between mental prosperity and actual wellbeing. By bringing issues to light and offering commonsense methodologies, people can find proactive ways to address both their psychological well-being concerns and balding issues.

There is a well-established association between stress and hair loss. Hair loss results from multiple factors, including environmental and genetic factors.

While acute stress boosts the immune system, chronic stress suppresses and over-activates Trusted Source the immune system, leading to inflammation.

Sustained and chronic stress can cause inflammation in or around the follicle, which can disrupt its mechanisms through endocrine and neuroimmune mediators like cortisol and corticotrophin-releasing hormones.

Hair growth involves three stages:

Anlagen:
the active phase where hair grows from the follicles
Cartagena:
phase involving the death or shrinkage (apoptosis) of the follicle at the base of the hair strand

telegenic:
resting phase in which the hair follicle is dormant and has no hair shaft growth. In this phase, the stem cells are quiescent, and hairs shed more easily
Stem cells found in hair follicles drive this hair cycle.

A 2021 rat study Trusted Source found that removing adrenal glands, which produce essential stress hormones in rats and humans, resulted in rapid hair regrowth cycles. Subjecting the rats to mild stress for weeks resulted in increased stress hormone (corticosterone) levels and reduced hair growth.

The hair follicles were also in an extended resting phase (telegenic). To add, corticosterone also prevents the cluster of cells (dermal papilla) beneath the stem cells from secreting a molecule that activates the hair follicle stem cells.

Learn more about thinning hair.

Types of stress-related hair loss

Three types of stress-related hair loss are associated with extreme stress levels.

telegenic effluvium

telegenic effluvium is the excessive hair shedding of resting (telegenic) hair. In a typical person's scalp, 85% of hair Trusted Source is antigen, while 15% is telegenic. Some stressors induce 70% of antigen hair into telegenic, leading to hair loss.

According to the American Academy of Dermatology (AAD), telegenic effluvium or excessive hair shedding is common among people who experience extreme stress. Common stressors include:

excessive weight loss
giving birth
major life stressors, such as job loss, divorce, death

high fever
recovering from an illness
stopping taking birth control pills

Other inducing factors include:

systemic diseases
major surgeries
drugs
nutritional deficiencies
This shedding usually occurs 3 months Trusted Source after the stressor. It is usually self-limiting and lasts for about 6 months. Chronic telegenic effluvium exceeds 6 months.

Alopecia aerate

Alopecia aerate involves the body's immune system attacking the hair follicles in the antigen phase, which forces them to the cartage phase. Because the stem cells in the follicles are not destroyed, the hair follicles continue to regenerate and continue cycling.

Clinically, it presents as small bald patches on the scalp or around the body and may lead to total loss of scalp or body hair.

Environmental triggers play a significant role in its development. Some also consider stressful life events as significant factors that trigger the condition. There is evidence to show that genetic factors may also play a role in the development of alopecia aerate.

Trichotillomania

Trichotillomania, or hair-pulling disorder, involves repeatedly pulling hair anywhere on the body. It is part of obsessive-compulsive disorder (OCD). A person with trichotillomania uses their hands, tweezers, or other devices to pull their hair.

The exact cause of trichotillomania remains unknown, but many people report the occurrence Trusted Source of a stressful event before the hair-pulling behavior. It may act as a person's coping mechanism to stress and anxiety.

Treatment for stress-related hair loss

Treatment for stress-related hair loss depends on the type of hair loss a person experiences.

telegenic effluvium

Acute telegenic effluvium is self-limiting Trusted Source and will typically resolve once the underlying cause is treated. Some research shows Trusted Source that the medication monoxide can help people with chronic telegenic effluvium. However, further research is needed to confirm the full effects it can have on hair shedding.

There is limited evidence on the effectiveness of treatments for alopecia aerate, but dermatologists prescribe topical corticosteroids as the first-line treatment for the condition.

Dermatologists may give topical corticosteroids to children 10 years old or younger and corticosteroid injections to individuals older than 10 years with patchy alopecia.

A dermatologist may prescribe topical immunotherapy in people with extensive alopecia (greater than 50% scalp hair loss). With this treatment, 74.6% of people Trusted Source with patchy alopecia experienced hair regrowth, and 54.4% of people with alopecia total is showed hair regrowth. However, 38.2% of people also experienced recurrence of their alopecia.

Trichotillomania

A healthcare team may use several treatment strategies to help manage trichotillomania. In children, conservative methods like using gloves or socks to cover the hands and cutting the hair short can help.

Habit reversal training, grounded in cognitive behavioral therapy (CBT), helps a person identify the cognitive distortions and the maladaptive behavior paired with them (hair-pulling) to change Trusted Source them.

Stress management tips

A number of stress management techniques Trusted Source can help a person cope with stress, including:

box breathing
guided imagery
progressive muscle relaxation
Below are other stress management tips that can help reduce stress and reduce the likelihood of hair loss due to stress Trusted Source:

eating nutritious, balanced meals
getting enough quality sleep
avoiding tobacco, alcohol, and substance use
taking time to do enjoyable activities
expressing worries and concerns to others
connecting with communities or faith-based organizations
trying meditating or spending time Trusted Source in nature
asking for professional help when necessary
Read more about stress-reduction strategies.

Other causes of hair loss

There are many other potential causes of hair loss. These include:

hereditary hair loss
cancer treatment
age
damaging hair care treatments
certain hairstyles
hormonal imbalance due to conditions like polycystic ovary syndrome (PCOS)
scalp infection
scalp psoriasis
medication
sexually transmitted infection (STI)
thyroid disease
friction
poison
nutrient deficiencies, such as Trusted Source iron and vitamin D
Frequently asked questions

The following are some questions that people frequently ask about hair loss.

Will stress-related hair loss grow back?

Acute stress-related hair loss, called telegenic effluvium, tends to be self-limiting and resolves when the trigger is treated or removed.

What does hormonal hair loss look like?

The hair may look finer or thinner. It may also fall easily and grow slower than before.

What does stress hair loss look like?

Stress hair loss, or telegenic effluvium, looks like hair falling out quickly from combing, washing, or even just touching the hair. The hair on the scalp may be thinning, but the scalp looks healthy and does not have scales or rashes.

Summary

Hair loss can happen due to a variety of factors, including stress. There are several types of stress-related hair loss. Their results may range from short-term, self-limiting hair loss to permanent, irreversible hair loss. Identifying the cause of the hair loss and seeking appropriate treatment is essential.

Treatment depends on the underlying cause and may include lifestyle changes, medications, topical treatments, and immunotherapy. Stress management techniques, such as deep breathing, can also help manage stress and decrease the risk of hair loss.

Chapter 6

Scalp Health and Hair Loss

A sound scalp is the establishment for delectable locks, yet it frequently gets neglected in hair care schedules. Scalp wellbeing assumes a urgent part in hair development and can essentially influence going bald examples. This guide expects to dive into the complexities of scalp wellbeing, investigating its relationship with balding and giving noteworthy hints to keep up with ideal scalp conditions for energetic, strong hair.

I. Figuring out Scalp Life systems and Capability:

A. Design of the Scalp:

Epidermis, dermis, and subcutaneous tissue layers.
Hair follicles, sebaceous organs, and veins.
B. Scalp Usefulness:

Hair follicle sustenance and hair shaft creation.
Sebum creation and scalp dampness guideline.
II. Normal Scalp Conditions and Balding:

A. Dandruff and Seborrhea Dermatitis:

Causes, side effects, and effect on hair wellbeing.
Connection between parasitic excess and hair shedding.
B. Scalp Psoriasis:

Ongoing fiery condition influencing scalp skin.

Possible intensification of balding because of aggravation.

C. Folliculitis:

Disease or irritation of hair follicles.
Scarring alopecia as an outcome of serious folliculitis.

III. The Job of Scalp Wellbeing in Balding:

A. Interruption of the Hair Development Cycle:

Effect of scalp irritation on hair follicle movement.
Drawn out scalp conditions prompting hair scaling down.

B. Impact on Hair Follicle Imperativeness:

Decreased supplement conveyance to hair follicles.
Hindered oxygenation and hair development restraint.

IV. Advancing Scalp Wellbeing for Hair Development:

A. Delicate Purifying and Peeling:

Utilizing gentle shampoos and staying away from unforgiving synthetic substances.
Integrating scalp peeling to eliminate development and further develop flow.

B. Adjusting Scalp Dampness:

Hydrating the scalp with saturating medicines.
Trying not to over-wash to forestall unreasonable sebum creation.

C. Scalp Back rub and Animating Methods:

Advantages of scalp knead for flow and unwinding.

Integrating medicinal balms and scalp serums for added sustenance.

V. Wholesome Help for Scalp and Hair Wellbeing:

A. Fundamental Supplements for Hair Development:

Protein, nutrients (A, C, E), and minerals (iron, zinc).
Omega-3 unsaturated fats for scalp aggravation decrease.

B. Dietary Sources and Enhancements:

Integrating lean proteins, organic products, vegetables, and entire grains.
Thought of enhancements like biotin and collagen for hair support.

VI. Stress The executives and Scalp Wellbeing:

A. Effect of Weight on Scalp Conditions:

Stress-prompted irritation and cortisol rise.
Fuel of scalp conditions like dandruff and psoriasis.

B. Stress-Decrease Methods:

Care practices, yoga, and profound breathing activities.
Focusing on taking care of oneself and unwinding to lighten scalp strain.

VII. Proficient Treatment Choices for Scalp Wellbeing:

A. Dermatological Intercessions:

Doctor prescribed meds for scalp conditions (antifungals, corticosteroids).
Light treatment (phototherapy) for psoriasis and other provocative problems.

B. High level Scalp Medicines:

Scalp micro needling for upgraded retention of skin medicines.
PRP treatment to advance scalp revival and hair development.

VIII. Conclusion:

An all encompassing way to deal with scalp wellbeing is fundamental for forestalling going bald and cultivating ideal hair development. By tending to scalp conditions, supporting scalp imperativeness, and taking on a sustaining way of life, people can develop a climate helpful for flourishing hair. Focusing on scalp care upgrades stylish allure as well as advances generally prosperity and certainty.

IX. References:

[Rundown of logical examinations, dermatological assets, and respectable sources supporting the data introduced in the guide.]

This far reaching guide fills in as a guide for people looking to successfully focus on scalp wellbeing and battle going bald. By consolidating the suggested practices and medicines, peruses can set out on an excursion towards energetic, versatile hair and a better scalp.

Appearance and morphology of the hair is regarded as one of the divergent traits of human population. Hair has a distinct specialized anatomical structure. Hair fibers consist of three morphological components namely, the cuticle, the cortex, and the medulla. Layers of cuticle cells form the outer sheath of the hair fiber and are mainly responsible for the cosmetic properties of hair. The cuticle forms a protective barrier for the hair against the outside environment.[1] Mechanical properties of the hair are attributed to the cortex, which forms the bulk of the fiber. Hair is important trace evidence commonly encountered in almost all criminal cases. Forensic anthropologists routinely compare the morphological characteristics of the hair samples to determine a transfer.[2] However, many questions such as how can populations be analyzed and possibly distinguished based on the morphology and appearance of their hair still remain unanswered.

Malaysia is a place rich in ethnological diversity, and its population comprises of three major ethnic groups including Malay, Chinese, and Indians, and other groups with diverse cultural backgrounds.[3]

In recent years, literature has approved that ethnicity and race are important factors to consider in the clinical presentation, management, and treatment of skin and hair disorders. Taking care of scalp is essential because it determines the health and condition of the hair and also prevents the diseases of scalp and hair. In this study, we have tried to identify and focus on few factors that might affect scalp health such as environment, nutrition, and individual factors and factors which determine the health of hair such as personal hygiene, use of hair care products, and frequency of hairdressing and styling. Hence, the objectives of our study were to correlate race and hair types, to determine the awareness of hair care among Malaysian medical students, to distinguish the factors that affect the health of hair and scalp, and to find out ways to improve the scalp condition and hair care practices.

Go to:
METHODOLOGY
Sample size

We did a cross-sectional study based on random sampling method for which ethical clearance was obtained from the Institutional Ethics Committee (IEC 820/2015) before the study, and the students gave their informed consent before taking part in this study. A total of 240 medical undergraduate students comprising of 120 male students and 120 female students aged 17–19 years were chosen randomly to participate in the study. These students belonged to three different Malaysian ethnic races, i.e., Malay (80 students), Chinese (80 students), and Malaysian Indians (80 students), and their participation was purely on voluntary basis. The period of study was 5 months. Students who did not wish to take part in the study, students with diseases of scalp, wounds of scalp, and students who had complaints of permanent hair loss were excluded from the study.

Data collection

Questionnaires were used in the study. This questionnaire constituted of 15 close-ended questions which were framed based on the objectives of our study and included questions on scalp and hair condition, hair care practices, and hairstyling methods of students. It also included student's demographic data. The questionnaire was then validated by academic faculty and ethics committee. This questionnaire was then distributed to the students in their classroom, and they were instructed to fill in their responses. These responses were then analyzed.

Data analysis

All the data which were obtained after evaluating the questionnaires were segregated according to the ethnic race and gender. The procured data were compiled, organized, and analyzed by using percentage statistics. The results obtained were represented as graphs using Microsoft Excel 2013.

Go to:
RESULTS

Our first observation was regarding the scalp condition of students. We found that Chinese students had comparatively healthier scalp (75% male, 92.5% female) without dandruff when compared to Malay and Indian students [Graph 1]. To compare their hair texture, we grouped the hair texture into four types: (1) silky hair, (2) dry and rough hair, (3) oily hair, and (4) hair with split ends and breakages. Among males, most Chinese (57.5%) and Indians (55%) had silky type of hair while Malay males had dry, rough hair (45%) and silky hair (45%). Only 10% of Indian male had oily hair while split ends and breakages were seen mostly in Malay males (10%). Among the females, generally silky hair was predominant (Chinese 35%, Malay 35%, Indians 32.5%). Dry and rough hair was seen more in Malay females (45%), and hair with split ends and breakages was seen mostly in Indian females (25%) followed by Chinese (17.5%) and Malay (10%) [Graph 2]. This shows that Chinese mostly own silky hair while Malay showed a higher percentage of rough and dry hair while Indians had a mix of silky and dry hair. Graying of hair was seen in a very less percentage of students, and it was seen mostly among female students [Graph 3]. In recent years, the trend mostly seen among teenagers is hair coloring and hairstyling. When we checked this trend among our study population, we found that among Chinese, 40% males and 52.5% females colored their hair. Among Malay, only females (22.5%) colored their hair. Among Indians also, this trend of coloring hair was slightly less for males as 12.5% males and 57.5% females colored their hair [Graph 4]. When these students were asked regarding their hair condition, male students felt that hair coloring did not worsen their hair condition (68%) while female students felt that it did affect their hair condition (75%). Hairstyling such as straightening and curling were mostly done by female students, and among them, Indians (50%) and Chinese (37.5%) predominantly did hair straightening and 10% Indians and 17.5% Chinese did hair curling. It was seen that most Malay females did not do any hairstyling methods (57.5%) [Graph 5]. When these students were asked regarding their hair condition, Chinese (66.7%) and Malay females (53%) feel that hairstyling worsened their hair condition while Indian females felt that it did not worsen their hair condition (52%). When asked regarding the frequency with which students changed their pillow covers, it was seen that majority of them changed their pillow covers once in a month (about 60%) while a few changed the covers twice a month (about 25%) and rest once in every 6 months. Our next important observation was regarding hair care practices. Among males, most of them washed their hairs twice a day (65.8%), and the rest (34.2%) washed their hair once a day. Among females, Chinese (65%) and Malay (50%) washed their hairs once in a day while Indian females mostly washed their hair once in 2 days (65%) [Graph 6]. Regarding hair care products used by the students, we found that most male students use only shampoo while very few also use shampoo and conditioner. Among females, most of them used shampoo and conditioner for hair wash. We also observed that Indian males (10%) and females (25%) used coconut oil along with shampoo while students of other two races did not use coconut oil [Graph 7]. We asked students if they face any type of stress to see if this relates to hair loss and hair condition. We found that most of the students face examination-related stress and most Chinese and Malay students also face dietary stress [Graph 8].

Chapter 7

Hairstyling Practices and Hair Damage

Hair styling is a fundamental piece of self-articulation and individual prepping for some people. Notwithstanding, over the top or ill-advised styling practices can prompt different types of hair harm, including breakage, split finishes, and even going bald. This exhaustive aide means to dig into the science behind hair styling, investigating normal practices, the effect of styling items, and systems to forestall and relieve hair harm.

I. Understanding Hair Design and Synthesis:

A. Life structures of the Hair Shaft:

Fingernail skin, cortex, and medulla layers.
Significance of keratin protein in hair design and strength.

B. Factors Affecting Hair Wellbeing:

Hereditary inclination to hair attributes.
Ecological factors like mugginess and UV openness.

II. Normal Hair Styling Practices:

A. Heat Styling:

Blow-drying, level pressing, and twisting procedures.
Effect of high temperatures on hair protein denaturation and dampness misfortune.

B. Substance Medicines:

Hair shading, perming, and loosening up strategies.
Compound fixings and their consequences for hair construction and honesty.

C. Mechanical Pressure:

Tight hairdos (pig tails, meshes) and hair adornments.
Contact from brushing and brushing rehearses.

III. Understanding Hair Harm:

A. Sorts of Hair Harm:

Warm Harm: Heat-incited protein corruption and dampness misfortune.
Substance Harm: Disturbance of hair bonds and fingernail skin trustworthiness.
Mechanical Harm: Actual injury prompting breakage and split closes.

B. Combined Harm Over the long haul:

Ongoing openness to styling practices and items.
Moderate decay of hair wellbeing and appearance.

IV. Effect of Styling Items:

A. Hair Styling Items:

Hair splashes, gels, mousses, and serums.
Fixings like alcohols, silicones, and polymers.

B. Hair Care Items:

Shampoos, conditioners, and medicines.
Details focusing on unambiguous hair types and concerns.

V. Forestalling Hair Harm:

A. Heat Styling Procedures:

Utilizing heat protectant items prior to styling.
Changing temperature settings and limiting openness time.

B. Restricting Substance Openness:

Picking delicate details and expert administrations.
Following appropriate application and post-treatment care rules.

C. Embracing Delicate Hair Care Practices:

Utilizing wide-toothed brushes and delicate shuddered brushes.
Keeping away from forceful towel drying and unnecessary control.

VI. Feeding and Fixing Harmed Hair:

A. Hydrating Medicines:

Profound molding veils and leave-in conditioners.
Integrating normal oils (argan, coconut) for dampness renewal.

B. Protein Recreation:

Protein-rich medicines to reinforce hair structure.
Hydrolyzed keratin and collagen details for fix.

VII. Proficient Mediations for Hair Fix:

A. Salon Medicines:

Protein medicines and keratin smoothing methodology.
Dampness imbuement treatments and scalp medicines.

B. Trim and Rebuilding:

Ordinary trims to eliminate split closes and forestall further harm.
Hair rebuilding choices for serious harm or going bald worries.

VIII. Embracing Sound Styling Practices:

A. Styling Choices:

Embracing air-drying and sans heat styling techniques.
Trying different things with defensive styles and embellishments.

B. Focusing on Hair Wellbeing:

Offsetting styling wants with hair care needs.
Putting resources into quality devices and items for long haul hair wellbeing.

IX. Conclusion:

Understanding the effect of hair styling practices and items on hair wellbeing is fundamental for keeping up with dynamic, tough locks. By taking on delicate styling procedures, limiting compound openness, and focusing on hair care, people can forestall and alleviate harm, guaranteeing their hair stays wonderful and smart long into the future.

X. References:

[Rundown of logical examinations, proficient assets, and trustworthy sources supporting the data introduced in the guide.]

This complete aide engages peruses to settle on informed conclusions about their hair styling works on, advancing better hair and improving generally certainty and prosperity. By consolidating the suggested methodologies, people can appreciate smart looks without compromising the wellbeing and honesty of their hair.
Changes that help prevent hair loss due to tight hairstyles
Anyone who frequently wears a tightly pulled hairstyle can develop hair loss. In fact, there's actually a medical term for this type of hair loss. It's called traction alopecia (al-oh-pee-she).

You can reduce your risk of developing this type of hair loss by following these dermatologists' tips.

Avoid frequently wearing hairstyles that pull on your hair. Every once in a while, it's OK to wear your hair tightly pulled back, but you want to avoid wearing a tightly pulled hairstyle every day. The constant pulling can cause strands of your hair to break or fall out.

In time, the continuous pulling can damage your hair follicles. If you damage your hair follicles, your hair cannot grow back, so you develop permanent hair loss.

Hairstyles that constantly pull on your hair include:

Buns, ponytails, and up-dos that are tightly pulled
Cornrows
Dreadlocks
Hair extensions or weaves

Tightly braided hair

Wearing rollers to bed most of the time can also lead to hair loss, so dermatologists recommend styling your hair this way only on special occasions.
Avoid wearing hairstyles that pull on your hair
If you often wear your hair tightly pulled back, the first sign of hair loss may be broken hairs around your hairline or thinning hair where your hairstyle pulls tightly.

Woman with hair tightly pulled back

Loosen up the hairstyle. When you wear your hair pulled back, loosen the hairstyle a bit, especially around your hairline.

To reduce the constant pulling, you can:

Loosen braids, especially around your hairline
Wear a braided style for no longer than two to three months
Opt for thicker braids and dreadlocks
Loosen up your hairstyle
If your hairstyle feels painful, the style is too tight.

Change it up. Changing hairstyles can also help reduce the pull. Ideally, when you change styles, you want to give your hair a chance to recover. For example, after wearing cornrows, you may want to wear loose braids or go natural for a few months.

Cornrows

Cornrows, which pull at the roots of your hair, can cause hair loss. Wearing looser braids and changing your hairstyle after 2 or 3 months can prevent hair loss.

A small girl wearing a cornrow hairstyle
Follow these precautions when wearing a weave. Weaves and extensions are great way to add volume and length to your hair. To prevent them from causing hair loss, dermatologists recommend that you:

Wear them for short periods of time, as the pulling can increase your risk of developing traction alopecia
Remove them immediately, if they cause pain or irritate your scalp
Opt for sewn-in weaves rather than ones that use bonding glue
Have a professional relax your hair. A hairstylist who has training in chemical relaxers can chose the product that will achieve the results you want while minimizing the damage to your hair.

To find out whether your stylist has this training, ask. You should also ask what your stylist will do to help maintain the health of your hair.

Look for early signs of hair loss. If you wear hairstyles that pull tightly, take time every month to look for these early signs of hair loss:

Broken hairs around your forehead
A receding hairline
Patches of hair loss where your hair is pulled tightly
If you see any of the above, it's time to stop pulling on your hair so that your hair can regrow.

When the pulling continues, most people eventually notice that their hair stops growing. Where you once had hair, you'll see shiny, bald skin. When traction alopecia advances to this stage, your hair cannot grow back.

Change your hairstyle immediately if you notice any of the following problems. These are signs that your hairstyle or products could cause hair loss:

Pain from tightly pulled hair
Stinging on your scalp
Crusts on your scalp
Tenting (sections of your scalp are being pulled up like a tent)

When to see a board-certified dermatologist
If you have hair loss, it's never too early to see a board-certified dermatologist. People develop hair loss for many reasons. Your hairstyle may be the cause. It's also possible that something else is causing your hair loss, such as stress or hereditary hair loss. A board-certified dermatologist can get to the root of the problem.

Chapter 8
Medical Conditions and Hair Loss

Going bald is a typical concern influencing people of any age and sexes, with different basic ailments adding to its beginning. Understanding the connection between ailments and going bald is critical for exact analysis and successful treatment. This extensive aide means to investigate the assorted scope of ailments related with balding, including their causes, side effects, and accessible treatment procedures.

I. Outline of Hair Development Cycle and Balding:

A. Hair Development Stages:

Anlagen (development) stage.
Cartagena (temporary) stage.
telegenic (resting) stage.
Hexogen (shedding) stage.
B. Kinds of Balding:

Androgen etic alopecia (male/female example hair sparseness).
telegenic exhaust.
Alopecia aerate.
Scarring alopecia.

II. Ailments Related with Going bald:

A. Hormonal Problems:

Thyroid issues (hypothyroidism, hyperthyroidism).
Polycystic ovary disorder (PCOS).

Hormonal awkward nature (estrogen, testosterone).

B. Immune system Illnesses:

Alopecia aerate.
Lupus erythematous.
Scleroderma.

C. Dermatological Circumstances:

Scalp psoriasis.
Seborrhea dermatitis.
Lichen follicularis.

D. Nourishing Lacks:

Lack of iron frailty.
Lack of vitamin D.
Protein lack of healthy sustenance.

E. Ongoing Ailments:

Diabetes mellitus.
Persistent kidney infection.
Immune system hepatitis.

III. Grasping the Components of Going bald in Ailments:

A. Disturbance of Hair Development Cycle:

Hormonal changes influencing follicle action.
Insusceptible interceded annihilation of hair follicles.

B. Microcirculatory Changes:

Impeded blood stream to the scalp.
Decreased supplement and oxygen conveyance to hair follicles.

C. Incendiary Cycles:

Resistant reaction focusing on hair follicles.
Persistent irritation prompting hair scaling down.

IV. Perceiving Side effects and Indications of Ailments Causing Balding:

A. Changes in Hair Surface and Thickness:

Diminishing of hair shafts.
Expanded shedding or going bald patches.

B. Scalp Side effects:

Tingling, chipping, or redness.
Scalp delicacy or irritation.

C. Foundational Side effects:

Exhaustion and shortcoming.
Weight changes or feminine inconsistencies.

V. Determination and Assessment of Ailments Related with Balding:

A. Clinical History and Actual Assessment:

Point by point history of side effects and ailments.
Assessment of scalp, skin, and nails.

B. Lab Tests:

Thyroid capability tests.
Complete blood count (CBC) and serum ferritin levels.
Chemical boards (testosterone, estrogen).

C. Skin Biopsy and Imaging:

Scalp biopsy for histological investigation.
esperanto and trichoscopy for follicular appraisal.

VI. Therapy Procedures for Going bald Related with Ailments:

A. Clinical Administration:

Hormonal treatments (thyroid chemical substitution, oral contraceptives).
Immunosuppressive prescriptions (corticosteroids, methotrexate).
Skin medicines (monoxide, corticosteroid arrangements).

B. Healthful Supplementation:

Iron enhancements for weakness remedy.
Nutrient and mineral supplementation (vitamin D, biotin).

C. Way of life Alterations:

Stress the executives procedures.
Adjusted diet and ordinary activity.

VII. Proficient Intercessions for Serious Going bald Cases:

A. Hair Transplantation:

Follicular unit transplantation (FUT).
Follicular unit extraction (FUE).

B. Scalp Micro pigmentation (SMP):

Corrective inking to make the presence of hair thickness.
Reasonable for people with broad going bald or scarring alopecia.

VIII. Mental Help and Methods for dealing with especially difficult times:

A. Tending to Profound Effect:

Advising and support bunches for people encountering balding.
Empowering self-acknowledgment and certainty building works out.

B. Training and Strengthening:

Giving assets and data about going bald circumstances.
Engaging people to assume command over their treatment process.

IX. Conclusion:

Going bald can be a troubling side effect of hidden ailments, requiring intensive assessment and designated therapy draws near. By understanding the different scope of ailments related with going bald, medical services experts and people the same can team up to distinguish the underlying driver and execute powerful administration techniques. Through a comprehensive methodology including clinical mediation, way of life changes, and mental help, people can explore their going bald excursion with certainty and versatility.

X. References:

[Rundown of logical examinations, clinical diaries, and legitimate sources supporting the data introduced in the guide.]

This complete aide fills in as an important asset for people looking to figure out the mind boggling connection between ailments and balding. By bringing issues to light and giving noteworthy bits of knowledge, it engages peruses to make proactive strides towards analysis, treatment, and all encompassing prosperity even with going bald difficulties

Many conditions can bring on hair loss. Some of the most common are pregnancy, thyroid disorders, and anemia. Others include:

Ringworm, which spreads from person to person and can cause bald spots

Other skin conditions such as psoriasis and seborrhea dermatitis

Scalp infections

Sexually transmitted infections

High fever

An autoimmune disease called alopecia aerate, in which your own immune system attacks your follicles, leaving round bald patches

Scarring alopecia, most often seen in Black women, in which hair starts falling out from the middle of the scalp and fans out, leaving areas of the scalp smooth and shiny

Diabetes

Sometimes hair loss is a sign of a condition called hyperandrogenism, which happens when your body makes too many androgens (male hormones). In women and others with female reproductive organs, its most common cause is polycystic ovary syndrome (PCOS). Along with hair loss, other signs of PCOS include weight gain, acne, and irregular periods. It's one of the most common causes of infertility.

Certain medications can lead to hair loss in some people, too. They include birth control pills, blood thinners, and some steroids.

Stress

You can have hair loss as a result of physical stress, like when you give birth or have surgery, or intense emotional stress, like a death in the family, divorce, or unemployment. Hair loss can happen a couple of weeks to 6 months after any stressful experience.

RELATED:
Men's Hair Loss: Here's What to Do

This type of hair loss is usually temporary. Once the stress goes away, your hair may get back to normal in 6-9 months.

Trichotillomania

Sometimes, people react to stress by plucking hairs from their head, eyebrows, and other places on their body. This disorder is called trichotillomania. It's a way for some people to ease tension, frustration, and other uncomfortable feelings. If you're embarrassed by a need to pull your hair or can't stop pulling it, talk to your doctor. Symptoms can get worse over time. Once you stop plucking hairs, they'll probably regrow.

Diet And Nutrition

If you lose more than 15 pounds in a short time, you might lose some of your hair as your body reacts to the shock. Other reasons for hair loss include:

A shortage of iron, protein, or other nutrients
Too much vitamin A (usually from supplements)
A shortage of vitamin D (which you can correct by taking supplements)
Anorexia (severely restricting yourself from food) or bulimia (throwing up on purpose after eating)
Hormones
Several types of hormonal changes can lead to hair loss. They include:

Menopause.

 You can lose hair during menopause as your estrogen and progesterone levels drop. Also, because hair follicles shrink during this time, your hair might be thinner, fall out easier, and grow more slowly.

 If you're going through menopause, talk to your doctor about ways to maintain or regrow your hair.

Pregnancy and childbirth. Pregnancy, and especially giving birth, can lead to hair loss. You're most likely to see hair loss about 3 months after giving birth. That's because your estrogen levels drop after childbirth. Your hair may fall out in clumps. If you're losing hair while pregnant, ask your doctor if you might have a dietary deficiency.

Hair usually regrows when your hormones get back to normal. Your hair can regain its usual fullness 6 to 9 months after childbirth.

Age. Hormonal changes as you age can cause hair loss. Hair growth naturally slows with age, so you may notice thinning. Some follicles eventually stop growing hair. If you think you have age-related hair loss, talk to your doctor about treatment early on.

RELATED:
Video: What Men Should Know About Hair Loss

Hair Loss In Transgender and No binary People
Anyone can have androgen etic alopecia (pattern baldness). These hair changes can make it hard to maintain how you want to look, especially if you're transgender or no binary (which means you don't identify as fully male or female). You may want to shift where hair grows (or doesn't) to reflect your affirmed gender.

Taking hormones can change hair growth all over your body. Masculinizing hormone therapy (taking testosterone) may cause hair loss within a year, and the effects aren't reversible if you stop hormone treatment.

Some people who take feminizing hormones, like estrogen or ant androgens, notice hair growth on their scalps (but the growth may not be significant, so you may need other treatments for hair loss). Scalp hair loss may slow down within 1-3 months, and you may have less facial and body hair after 6-12 months of treatment. Overall results could take 1-2 years.

Traction Alopecia

Traction alopecia is a type of hair loss that's brought on by the way you style your hair. Hairstyles like cornrows, braids, or tight ponytails can cause it. Some signs of traction alopecia include hair loss in patches where the hair was pulled and shorter strands of hair near the forehead.

Other styling habits that can lead to breakage and thinning hair include:

High heat from blow dryers or flat irons

Harsh chemicals from bleach, perms, or other products
Tightly pulled hair from clips, bands, or pins
Over-shampooing or brushing and combing too much, especially when your hair is wet
With most of these issues, your hair can grow back. But if your follicles become damaged, the hair loss may be permanent. See your dermatologist if you notice this type of hair loss. The sooner you start treatment, the better the chances for hair regrowth.

Diagnosis

When you see a doctor to see what's causing your hair loss, they'll probably start with a physical exam and ask about your diet, family history, and medical history. They may ask whether any of your relatives have hair loss.

RELATED:
Video: What Men Should Know About Hair Loss

They can also do tests such as:

Blood tests. This helps them look for conditions like thyroid problems or low iron.

Light microscopy.
 Your doctor may use a lighted microscope to look for any hair shaft disorders.

Pull test.
 For this test, they gently pull on a chunk of your hair to see how many strands come out.

Scalp exam.
Looking at your scalp lets your doctor check for any infections or swelling and see where your hair's falling out.

Biopsy.
 Your doctor gently scrapes skin samples from your scalp and sends them to a lab for testing.

How Is Female Hair Loss Treated?
The treatment for hair loss depends on what's causing it. If a medical condition is the cause, treating that

condition should help with the hair loss. If it's caused by a medication, your doctor can change your drug or the dosage.

Treatments may include:

Medications. Monoxide (Rogaine) is a topical medication (the type you apply to your scalp) approved by the FDA for female pattern hair loss. It's is available over the counter as 2% and 5% solutions. It takes about 6-12 months of this once-daily use foam treatment to see results.

The medication works by prolonging the growth phase of hair, giving your hair more time to grow out.

If you're pregnant, planning to become pregnant, or breastfeeding, ask your doctor before taking monoxide. It may be harmful to your unborn baby and can pass through breast milk to a nursing infant.

Spironolactone is another medication your doctor may prescribe for hair regrowth and to keep hair loss from getting worse. It stops the action of male hormones called androgens.

Supplements. If you have a deficiency, your doctor may suggest multivitamins or supplements like iron and biotin. Don't take any supplement before checking with your doctor. They may interact with other medications or supplements you take.

Hair transplants.
 This is a procedure in which your doctor removes hair from a part of your scalp where hair growth is full and implants it into an area where hair is thinning.

Chapter 9

Natural Remedies and Hair Growth

Normal cures have been used for a really long time to advance hair development and keep up with scalp wellbeing. From home grown concentrates to medicinal ointments, nature offers a plenty of fixings with implied benefits for hair care. This complete aide means to investigate the science behind normal solutions for hair development, digging into their viability, security, and reasonable applications.

I. Understanding the Hair Development Cycle:

A. Hair Development Cycle Outline:

Anlagen (development) stage.
Cartagena (momentary) stage.
telegenic (resting) stage.
Hexogen (shedding) stage.
B. Factors Affecting Hair Development:

Hereditary qualities and hormonal equilibrium.
Dietary status and scalp wellbeing.

II. Famous Normal Solutions for Hair Development:

A. Medicinal balms:

Rosemary oil: Animates hair follicles and further develops course.
Lavender oil: Advances hair development and diminishes pressure instigated going bald.

Peppermint oil: Increments scalp flow and may improve hair thickness.

B. Natural Concentrates:

Saw palmetto: Blocks DHT, a chemical related with going bald.

Ginseng: Further develops hair follicle expansion and animates development.

Aloe Vera:

Calms the scalp and advances hair development.

C. Supplement Rich Oils:

Coconut oil: Saturates the scalp and diminishes protein misfortune in hair.

Argon oil

: Sustains hair follicles and improves sparkle.

Castor oil: Contains ricin oleic corrosive, which might advance hair development.

III. The Science Behind Normal Solutions for Hair Development:

A. Components of Activity:

Animating blood flow to the scalp.

Obstructing catalysts related with going bald (e.g., 5-alpha-reductase).

Giving fundamental supplements to hair follicle wellbeing.

B. Research Proof:

Clinical investigations assessing the viability of natural concentrates and rejuvenating oils.

Creature and research center examinations explaining the atomic instruments of regular cures.

IV. Down to earth Applications and Utilization Tips:

A. Effective Application:

Weakening medicinal balms with transporter oils for scalp kneads.
Making Do-It-Yourself hair covers with home grown concentrates and supplement rich oils.

B. Scalp Back rub Methods:

Delicate roundabout movements to further develop blood stream and item assimilation.
Integrating scalp knead into ordinary hair care schedules.

V. Joining Regular Cures with Way of life Changes:

A. Solid Eating regimen:

Integrating supplement thick food varieties for ideal hair development.
Hydration and satisfactory protein consumption for hair follicle wellbeing.

B. Stress The executives:

Rehearsing unwinding methods like contemplation and profound relaxing.
Focusing on taking care of oneself to decrease pressure related balding.

VI. Security Contemplations and Expected Dangers:

A. Unfavorably susceptible Responses:

Fix testing rejuvenating ointments and home grown separates before full application.
Weakening powerful fixings to limit skin awareness.

B. Collaboration with Drugs:

Conference with a medical care proficient, particularly for people taking drugs.
Consciousness of possible communications between normal cures and recommended drugs.

VII. Setting Sensible Assumptions:

A. Continuous Outcomes:

Understanding that regular cures might require some investment to show perceptible impacts.
Consistency and persistence are vital to accomplishing wanted results.

B. Individual Changeability:

Perceiving that reactions to normal cures might change among people.
Changing plans and use in light of individual experience and inclinations.

VIII. Conclusion:

Regular cures offer promising potential for advancing hair development and keeping up with scalp wellbeing, drawing upon the rich abundance of botanicals and supplement rich oils. By understanding the science behind these cures, people can outfit their advantages successfully and coordinate them into all encompassing hair care schedules. With legitimate utilization, wellbeing safeguards, and sensible assumptions, normal cures can be important partners in accomplishing energetic, solid hair.

IX. References:

[Rundown of logical examinations, clinical preliminaries, and trustworthy sources supporting the data introduced in the guide.]

This exhaustive aide fills in as a significant asset for people looking for normal answers for hair development and scalp wellbeing. By integrating proof based practices and security contemplations, peruses can set out on an excursion towards supporting their hair with the abundance of nature, cultivating versatility and imperativeness from root to tip.

Chapter 10
Professional Treatments and Solutions

Going bald can fundamentally affect a singular's confidence and certainty, inciting numerous to look for proficient medicines and arrangements. From clinical intercessions to cutting edge restorative methodology, there are different choices accessible to address various sorts and levels of going bald. This far reaching guide expects to investigate the domain of expert going bald medicines, covering their systems of activity, viability, and contemplations for people looking for answers for their balding worries.

I. Figuring out the Range of Balding:

A. Kinds of Balding:

Androgen etic alopecia (male and female example hair loss).
telegenic exhaust.
Alopecia aerate.
Scarring alopecia.

B. Evaluating and Characterization:

Norwood-Hamilton scale for male example hairlessness.
Ludwig scale for female example balding.
Seriousness appraisal in view of hair thickness and scalp inclusion.

II. Clinical Intercessions for Balding:

A. Oral Prescriptions:
Finasteride (Prophecies):
 Restrains the change of testosterone to dihydrotestosterone (DHT) to forestall hair scaling down.
Dutasteride:
 Another 5-alpha-reductase inhibitor involved off-mark for going bald treatment.
Spironolactone: Against androgen prescription recommended off-name for female example going bald.
B. Skin Medicines:

Monoxide (Rogaine): Vasodilator that advances hair development by expanding the antigen period of the hair development cycle.
Effective Finasteride: Option in contrast to oral Finasteride with confined consequences for the scalp.
Blend treatments: Monoxide joined with enemies of androgens or development factors for improved viability.
C. Injectable Medicines:

Platelet-rich plasma (PRP) treatment: Concentrated platelets from the patient's blood infused into the scalp to animate hair development.
Undifferentiated cell treatment: Using undifferentiated cells to recover hair follicles and advance hair development.

III. Careful Answers for Hair Rebuilding:

A. Follicular Unit Transplantation (FUT):

Strip reaping procedure including the expulsion of a giver take from the scalp.
Canalization of follicular units under a magnifying lens for transplantation into beneficiary destinations.

B. Follicular Unit Extraction (FUE):

Individual follicular units reaped straightforwardly from the scalp utilizing a punch device.
Insignificantly obtrusive methodology with no straight scar, reasonable for more modest areas of transplantation.

C. Automated Hair Transplantation:

Robotized follicular unit extraction involving automated innovation for exact and productive gathering.
Benefits incorporate decreased technique time and expanded precision.
IV. High level Corrective Methodology for Hair Improvement:

A. Scalp Micro pigmentation (SMP):

Corrective inking method to reproduce the presence of hair follicles on the scalp.
Appropriate for people with broad balding or scarring alopecia.

B. Hair Frameworks and Hairpieces:

Uniquely designed hairpieces and hairpieces to cover thinning up top regions.

Regular looking and adjustable choices for people looking for non-careful arrangements.

V. Contemplations for Picking Proficient Balding Medicines:

A. Individual Balding Profile:

Type and seriousness of going bald.
Patient inclinations and assumptions.

B. Clinical History and Contraindications:

Prior ailments and prescriptions.
Sensitivities or aversions to treatment parts.

C. Cost and Long haul Support:

Beginning speculation and progressing support costs.
Obligation to follow-up arrangements and treatment regimens.

VI. Consolidating Medicines for Ideal Outcomes:

A. Blend Treatment Approaches:

Oral prescriptions joined with skin medicines for synergistic impacts.
Careful hair rebuilding followed by support with clinical or corrective mediations.

B. Customized Treatment Plans:

Custom fitted methodologies in view of individual requirements and treatment reactions.
Progressive heightening or change of medicines on a case by case basis

VII. Tending to Mental Effect and Backing Needs:

A. Advising and Instruction:

Giving data about treatment choices and anticipated results.
Tending to worries about self-perception and confidence.

B. Support Gatherings and Companion Organizations:

Interfacing people with others encountering comparable difficulties.
Peer support and imparted encounters in adapting to balding.

VIII. Conclusion:

Proficient going bald therapies offer assorted choices for people looking to address their going bald worries, going from clinical mediations to cutting edge restorative methodology. By figuring out the components of activity, viability, and contemplations for treatment determination, people can pursue informed choices and leave on an excursion towards hair rebuilding and reestablished certainty. With the direction of gifted experts and an extensive way to deal with treatment, the mission for sound, energetic hair becomes feasible for some.

IX. References:

[Rundown of logical examinations, clinical preliminaries, and legitimate sources supporting the data introduced in the guide.]

This complete aide fills in as an important asset for people thinking about proficient going bald medicines and arrangements. By giving experiences into accessible choices, contemplations, and backing procedures, it engages peruses to explore their balding excursion with certainty and informed direction.